Essentials of Cardiovascular Training

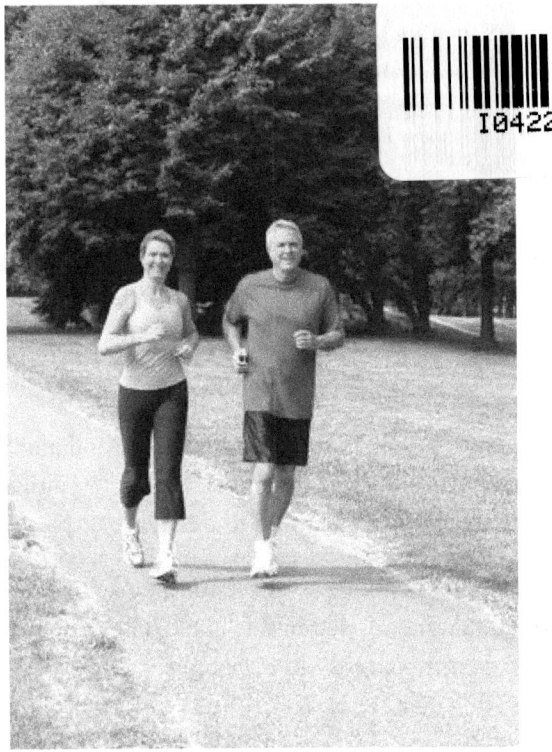

Health Learning Series

M. Usman

Mendon Cottage Books

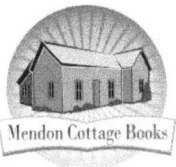

JD-Biz Publishing

Disclaimer

The information is this book is provided for informational purposes only. It is not intended to be used and medical advice or a substitute for proper medical treatment by a qualified health care provider. The information is believed to be accurate as presented based on research by the author.

The contents have not been evaluated by the U.S. Food and Drug Administration or any other Government or Health Organization and the contents in this book are not to be used to treat cure or prevent disease.

The author or publisher is not responsible for the use or safety of any diet, procedure or treatment mentioned in this book. The author or publisher is not responsible for errors or omissions that may exist.

Warning

The Book is for informational purposes only and before taking on any diet, treatment or medical procedure, it is recommended to consult with your primary health care provider.

Our books are available at

1. Amazon.com
2. Barnes and Noble
3. Itunes
4. Kobo
5. Smashwords
6. Google Play Books

Table of Contents

Preface

Diseases associated with the cardiovascular system are one of the leading causes of mortality in the US. They account for almost 50 percent of all the recorded deaths that occur every year and moreover, affect the lives of 14 million people. This number includes those with chest pain, known as angina pectoris, as well as people who have defects in their hearts which result in ineffective pumping of the blood. This ultimately leads to the tissues getting inadequate blood. Almost 1.5 million Americans suffer from heart attacks each year and approximately $1/3^{rd}$ of these perish. Each year almost 700,000 patients who have heart disease, choose the surgery option and undergo by-pass surgery to recover from their condition.

It must be pondered over that surgery is not the answer to every disease, especially this one. There are a lot of other options that can naturally do the same job, and one of these options is cardio training. The book will enlighten you about the whole concept of cardiovascular training and how it benefits the body. Plus, it packs a training program which can help you enormously if you're a person who plans to get better cardiovascular health.

The next section will deal with the importance of cardiovascular training.

Getting Started

Chapter # 1: Introduction

Over the last 40 years, several medical and scientific reports have analyzed the relationship between the level of physical activity and a person's cardiovascular health. Organizations like the Centers for Disease Control & Prevention, American Heart Association, and American College of Sports medicine have convened expert panels that have found scientific linkage between physical activity and a person's cardiovascular health. These panels, along with the 1996 US Surgeon Report, have found concrete evidence that fit, or more precisely active, individuals have a lesser chance of developing heart diseases compared to people who spend most of the time sitting or idle. Even if a heart disease does develop in active people, it develops due to old age and is of very much low intensity. Studies have also found that physical activity is not only helpful in protecting the cardiovascular system, but also proves beneficial with a host of other problems like osteoporosis, colon cancer, hypertension, diabetes, etc.

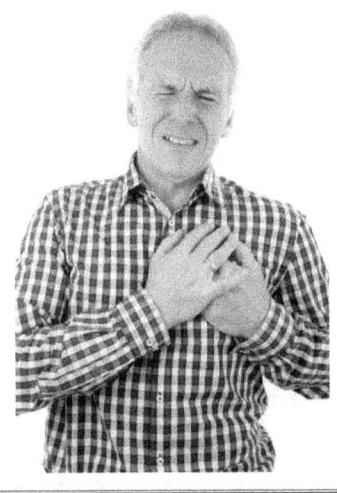

Comparatively, there is still a higher occurrence of cardiovascular disease when individuals are found to put a halt to their physical movements. Even the chance of midlife increases when a person engages in exercise, through change in activities, this is often linked with a decrease in the risk of mortality. But the sad fact is that despite of all these evidences and resources, US nationals still rest carelessly and ignorantly. Less than a third of these individuals meet the lowest requirement there is for physical activity, as outlined by the various institutions stated in the opening paragraph.

Chapter # 2: Benefits and Risks

Cardiovascular disease has a total of five risk factors:

1. A sedentary lifestyle

2. High blood pressure

3. Abnormal level of lipids

4. Obesity

5. Smoking

These factors have been outlined by the American Health Association and carry great importance. Many scientific researchers have suggested that reduction in the stated risk factors can drastically decrease the risk associated with cardiovascular disease like having a heart attack or experiencing a cardiac event, e.g. a stroke. It also reduces the possibility for the patient undergoing a by-pass surgery also known as the re-vascularization procedure.

Regular fitness activities, like exercise, can positively affect the established risk of these factors that lead to cardiovascular disease. For example, exercise can lead to a reduction in weight, which would lead to controllable blood pressure. Exercise can also reduce the amount of bad cholesterol, also known as LDL, in the blood and increase the level of good cholesterol, also called HDL cholesterol, in the blood. For patients who have diabetes, everyday activity enhances the body's skills in dealing with insulin, which controls the level of glucose streaming in the blood. Still, it must be noted that even though the effect of an exercise program that lasts shortly, is not very long-lasting, regular and moderate amounts of exercise can decrease the overall risk of cardiovascular disease, especially when it is performed in conjunction with lifestyle alterations like quitting cigarettes.

Exercise has a lot of physiological benefits as well and 2 examples of such improvements are a gain in muscular strength, as well as enhancement in function. Exercise allows the body to increase its input of oxygen, which leads to improved function of the whole body. As a person's ability to use oxygen is improved, and it leads to a direct improvement in his/her performance in day-to-day activities. This is especially vital for patients of heart disease who have a lower capacity to perform physical activities compared to those without any cardiovascular disease. Evidence is clearly stating that training can improve the blood vessel's capacity to expand as a result to hormonal release. This improved vascular function leads to better blood flow and provision of oxygen to the body's cells. Studies that compared the flexibility and muscle strength of subjects, before as well as after, an exercise routine found out that significant improvement was made in bone health as a result of exercise. Moreover, the likelihood of developing back pain also decreased.

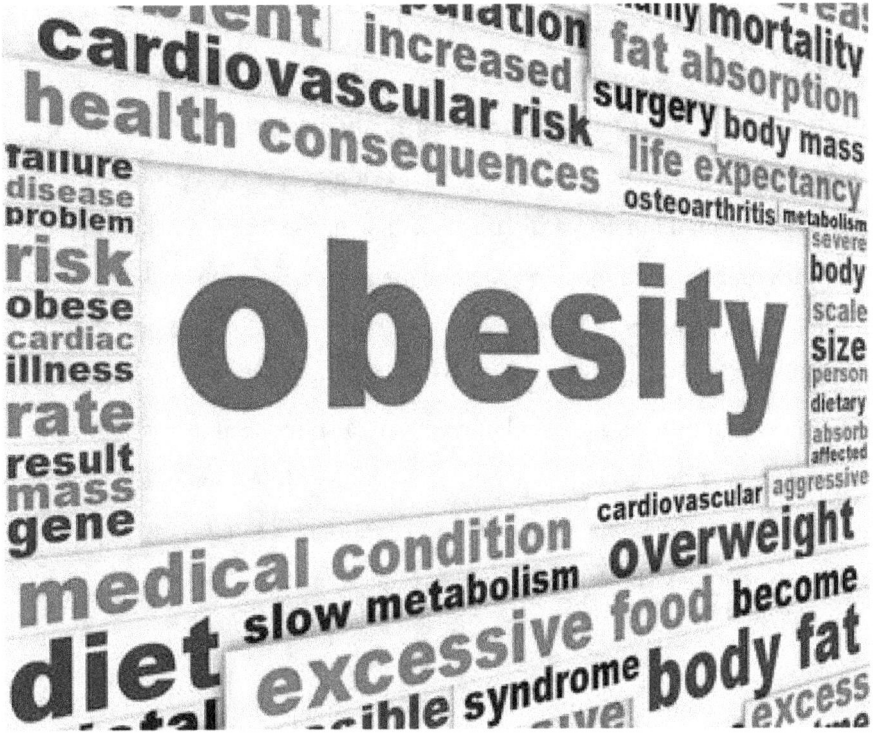

Patients who were freshly diagnosed with heart diseases participated in a physical program and reported an overall improvement in their lifestyle and cognitive qualities like confidence, stress levels, anxiety, etc. Important enough was the finding that patients of heart disease, who carried out physical activity, decreased their mortality risk by 20%. This was strong evidence as it suggested that there were alternatives to by-pass surgery. But before this chapter is finished, it must also be stated that even though scientists have found evidence of exercise's effectiveness in countering heart disease, it is still not enough to do so all by itself. Therefore, it requires the support of other entities, especially in patients who suffer from extreme cases.

Risks

The risk of cardiovascular diseases increases rapidly when a person carries out high intensity cardiovascular activity compared to when a person lives his/her routine life. This statement is especially important for patients of heart disease who have a general habit of leading a sedentary lifestyle. Estimates of high impact cardio diseases in exercise based rehabilitation facilities range from almost 1/100000 patient exercise hours to 1/300,000 patient exercise hours. Therefore, the method of rehabilitation through exercise has shown promising benefits, as serious conditions are rare. Did you know that rare cardiovascular events are also reduced in patients who are part of a cardiovascular program? Regardless of the type of exercise they carry out, cardio patients should always have four warning shots in their minds, which may show decline in heart function:

1. Recurring or new episodes of angina pain, which is pain in the chest, ache in the neck, or discomfort in the shoulders and back.

2. Lightheadedness

3. Rhythmic abnormalities with the heart

4. Dizziness

In such cases, a medical health provider should be contacted immediately with the training program discontinued. For patients with existing cardiovascular problems, a heart related incident could occur once in almost 62,000 hours and this is a significant number given the huge amount of people with cardiovascular diseases. At the same time, evidence from studies and reports has suggested that a sedentary person is almost at 50 times more risk than a normal exercising person with respect to cardiovascular diseases. Moreover, did you know that majority of heart attacks occur when a person is in resting state? Exercise is thus a very safe activity that can limit the chances of a heart attack, but nevertheless, it is best to check in with your doctor and keep yourself up to date with the latest warning signs.

Examples include:

- Maximal heart rate of 150 beats/minute,

- Resting heart rate should be 70 beats/minute,

- Training heart rate should be 118 beats/minute,

Although maximal heart rates are determined using a formula, such estimates are still not very real and can only truly be determined only by an exercise test.

Chapter # 3: How Much?

The Surgeon General's report on Physical Activity was released in 1996, which brought concrete evidence to the public's sight about the benefits of physical activity on one's health. This piece of evidence was a major marketer for exercise and played a key role in propelling exercise as a key adversary of heart disease or any cardiovascular disease. The study stated that activity was most promising when carried out at least 30 minutes every day on a moderate scale. However, this number proved too exhaustive for many and was soon brought down to 3 times a week for 12 consecutive weeks.

It was found that more exercise could benefit in a more pronounced manner, but if an individual withdrew from the program he/she would soon lose all the attained benefits. Aerobic exercise training sessions should be at least 30 minutes long, either consecutively or in 3x 10 minute portions. The intensity at which they should be carried out should be 85 percent of the person's heart rate. But, the heart rate that should be kept in mind is 10 beats/minute less than your maximum heart rate or that prescribed by a doctor. The last few lines are of vital importance, as you must have your doctor's approval before starting out on any exercise program.

Compared to other exercises, walking holds a significant edge. This is especially during the first few phases of an exercise program aimed to fight cardiovascular diseases. Training programs that focus on brisk walking can significantly improve the health risks that have been stated earlier on. Walking being an easy, tolerable exercise offers more advantages, as well as fewer problems, compared to running and jogging. It is an activity that requires almost little or no investment other than some good shoes that ensure comfort.

In clinically stable chronic patients, resistance training in addition to aerobic exercise can effectively increase muscle content in the body, which results in greater strength as well as endurance. The anatomical changes that are produced as a result of this also improve the cardiovascular risk factors and improve the heart's overall condition. Such training can also bring down the demand put forward by the cardiovascular system during leisure activities, which can increase the quality of a patient's personal life. Weight training programs that focus on a single set and are performed up to 3 times a week are far better than multi-set ones, as they provide almost the same benefits and are more time consuming. But any training program that you choose must target all the major muscle groups, namely shoulders, legs, chest, back, hips, etc. At least 10 exercises should be carried out to fulfill this compulsion. The set should allow 15 reps of medium intensity and should be carried out at least 3 times a week, along with changes in lifestyle habits.

The following is a table that compares different types of physical activities and their medicinal worth. Note that the recommended amount of physical activity is 5 – 7 half an hour sessions at an intensity of 3 to 6 Multiples of Resting Metabolic Rate (600 – 1200 calories burned a week).

	Activity	METs	Calories/Hour
1	Walking at 2 miles/hour	2.5	175
2	Walking at 3 miles per hour	3.5	245
3	Golf with cart	2.5	175

4	Golf without cart	4.9	340
5	Calisthenics	4.0	280
6	Gardening	4.4	310
7	Cycling	4.0	280
8	Cycling at moderate pace	5.7	400
9	Swimming slowly	4.5	315
10	Swimming at a fast pace	7.0	490
11	Climbing hills with no load	6.9	480
12	Climbing hills with 5 kg	7.5	525
13	Tennis single match	7.5	525
14	Tennis doubles match	6.0	420
15	Running 1 mile in 10 mins	10.2	710
16	Running 1 mile in 7.5 mins	13.2	930

It must also be noted that one does not need to be a marathon runner or an athlete if he/she is to derive a visible number of benefits from cardio workouts. The Surgeon General's Report was quite clear of this fact and in fact it suggested that a person gains maximum benefit when he/she shifts from sedentary life style to an energetic one. Reports have supported this finding and have shown that as the difference in activity gap shortens, less is gained by the person. One study that was carried out on US veterans showed that largest gains were made (mortality) by the lowest fitness groups and the successive lowest fitness group. The study was carried out on over 6000 men over a period of 6 years and compared parameters like the risk of death with the change in physical fitness. Did you know that adults who are at their least fitness levels have at least a 4.5 times higher mortality risk compared to adults who are actively fit? Surprisingly enough, the fact that any person's fitness level was a much more accurate death predictor compared to known risks like blood pressure, smoking, diabetes, cholesterol, etc. This study, in addition to dozens of others, underlines the statement that fitness, along with a level of physical activity, is a strong factor when it comes to determining the incidence of heart attacks or other cardiovascular diseases.

Optimum Program

Chapter # 1: Introduction

When performed correctly, cardiovascular exercises like cycling, running, or any activity that raises the heartbeat, can offer a wide variety of health benefits like reduced fat, increased metabolism, greater alertness, and better lifestyle. Furthermore, by exercising, the risk of disease drops and strokes, osteoporosis and diabetes are tackled. But these benefits can only be extracted if the exercise is performed correctly. If a person runs only for a few minutes and considers himself saved, then he/she is wrong and must know that effort must be put in, like a set of guidelines, if benefits are to be extracted truly. That's not the only drawback of wrong training; if a person trains on incorrect guidelines then he/she only risks making his conditions worse. Each person should therefore either train under the supervision of an expert or evaluate his/her condition first before making any decisions. Many scientific studies have brought down the number of factors that influence a training program to 4. They are:

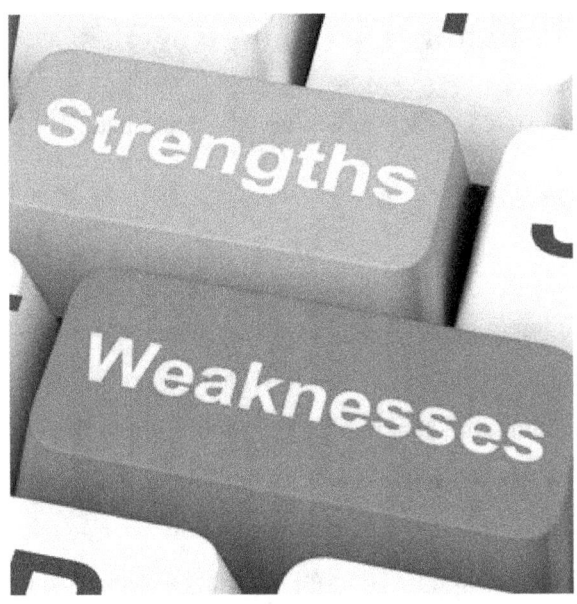

1. Goals – Is the goal of your whole workout to burn maximum fat or to improve the level of physical fitness you hold?

2. Age – As you age, the body's maximum heart rate decreases. Heart rate is a major argument that governs a person's training intensity and therefore must always be looked at with respect.

3. Conditioning – If you are already on some plan or in better shape, then you should exercise with greater intensity, as the curve starts to plateau as you gain more fitness.

4. Time – How much time do you have? For many people this is the most important factor and it probably should be, as it decides for how long and with what frequency you can engage in a physical program.

Chapter # 2: Putting Everything Together

The four factors stated earlier on will now be explained:

1. Intensity:

Almost every study and medical fitness expert recommends that any individual training to gain physical fitness, run at a rate that is 85% of what his/her heart allows. But sometimes, it is stated that running at a rate of up to 55 percent is much more beneficial when fat burning is the issue at hand. You must know that the statement of higher fat burning at lower intensity is a completely bogus one. Even though it is sometimes true that at low or moderate intensities more fat is burnt, the exact amount of cut fat is quite high when exercises are performed at higher intensities. The following example will make it easier for you to understand.

Two people who have similar body masses, as well as level of fitness, are made to run for almost the same length of time. The first person travels at a rate that is 40% of the maximum heart limit and burns calories close to 400; 70 percent of these calories comprise of fat while 30 percent are carbohydrates. The second person runs at 80 percent of what his/her heart allows, but runs a longer distance in the same length of time. He burns 700 calories out of which 50% are fat and 50% are carbohydrates. The person who travelled at an intensity level of 40 percent burned only 30 grams of fat while the other person who ran at 80 percent cut almost 39 grams of fat. Here's how:

- 70 percent of 400 kilocalories when divided by 9 kilocalories per gram give the amount of energy per gram.

- 50 percent of 700 kilocalories when divided by 9 kilocalories

While the first person who exercised at 40 percent maximum heart rate burned higher fat in percentage, the 2nd one, who had a higher pulse rate throughout the run, burned a far greater amount. The conclusion we get from this study is that if you run in between 60 – 80 percent of your heart rate, then you will achieve optimum physical fitness, burn more fat, and have a safer cardiovascular system. Moreover, even when you are resting you can burn fat due to higher metabolism which comes from exercising at a higher heart rate. An intensity of 60 to 80 percent should however, not be exceeded. If it is, then the body will substitute the fat with glycogen reserves which are carbohydrates stored in the body; the result will be less amount of fat burned and thus zero weight loss.

Therefore the **1st rule** is; the ideal level of intensity is *not low but high.*

2. Age:

Before going into the details, I just want to make one thing clear. Any person who is more than 35 years old and has not been involved in a physical activity for 1 year should first visit his/her doctor to make sure he/she is fit enough to perform. This is very necessary since you could be at risk of an illness that could get worse as a result of a training program. Having said that, you must also know that there are a few diseases which are very harmful during aerobic exercises.

Age is also a very important factor when it comes to evaluating the target heart rate, which is the rate at which a person must run to gain the maximum benefits. Generally speaking, the maximum heart rate decreases as a person ages, so it's different for individuals of various ages. You can make a rough guess of your max heart rate by the following equation:

(220 – Your age)

So for a 30-year-old person the heart rate is 190.

Therefore the **2nd rule** is; use the equation to find the target heart rate.

3. Level of Conditioning:

When you are new to a training program that features the cardiovascular system and have also avoided exercise for a long time, then you should start off with 60 percent intensity. This rule must be followed as the body can gradually adapt to change and if the stress exposed is too much to handle, then more harm may be done instead of good. And yes, you read it right; training is a form of stress. But if engaged in the correct fashion, it can be positive. It must also be known that heart is not the only part of the body that has to adapt to a training program, rather the body as a whole has to manage to get used to the new routine; the muscular system also has to adapt to the changes.

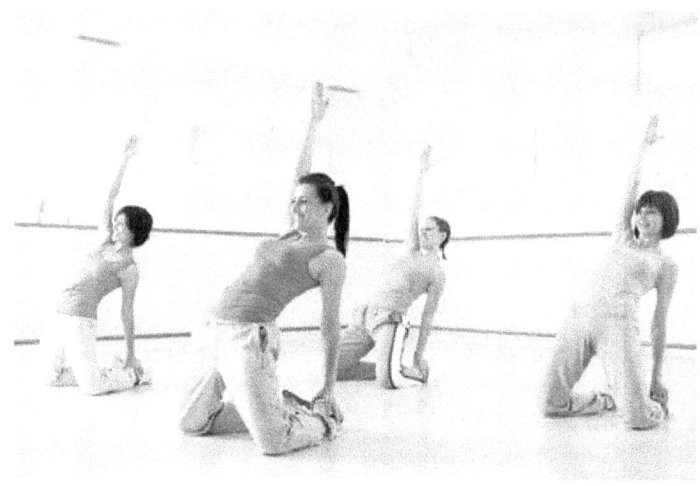

Now, even though starting off a cardio training routine may seem simple, it can get tricky at times and at no instance should you lose focus. If you want to increase the intensity, then do so, but gradually. A 5% increase per month can be enough to start with and you may increase the intensity from 60 percent to 75 percent, but not after that as it can get harmful as stated earlier on. Also note that it's best not to increase the intensity of exercise in the months when you skip the routine for 2 days in a row per week.

It is also wise to measure your resting pulse each day. The best time to do so is right after waking up or while you're still resting in bed, as at that time external factors like food, work, etc. do not play any role. If the training program is followed as explained, then after a few months of training you would start to notice a declining trend in the resting pulse.

The **3rd rule** is; when beginning with the routine, maintain an intensity of 60 percent of the maximum heart rate and gradually increase it with 5 percent additions.

4. Time:

For a person to find out the length of his/her cardiovascular session, he/she should first check in with his/her schedule to check out his availability. A rule of thumb for all starters is that one hour of training is mandatory every week. If you can't even take out this much time in the whole week, then it would be very hard for the body to show any progress. 60 minutes can then be easily broken down to smaller pieces and can become 20 minutes every alternate day. Having said that, 90 minutes a day should be your cap and you should not exceed it under any circumstances.

If you feel that the training sessions are long, e.g. 1 hour each day and they are putting a stress on your routine life, then you should consider resting every other day as the rest can help the body recharge itself. If your training program is carried out with the help of weights, then set one day for cardio while the other for weight training. For a training routine that packs both anaerobic as well as aerobic training, the best thing to do is include 1 complete rest day. Combine sufficient exercise with a healthy amount of nutrition and soon you'll start noticing the results; your glycogen reserves will soon fill up. The one day gap is necessary as it will not only decrease the risk of over-training, but will also fill up the body's glycogen reserves which would then effectively be used throughout the day. Many studies have shown that if a muscle is low on fuel, i.e. glycogen, an individual's routine can suffer sharply. A worst-case scenario would be working out at low glycogen reserves, as when he/she works out for any reason, e.g. gaining endurance, etc. he might actually burn more glycogen which will kick off a chain reaction extremely harmful for the body. This will improve neither the level of fitness nor the level of cardiovascular health in the person.

If shaving off extra fat is your number 1 priority then at least 4 cardio sessions a week should be on your training program. They can be effective at burning subcutaneous fat, which is stored under the skin. In order to achieve maximum fat burning, plan a program that contains both cardio and weight training. This way you will lose fat while at the same time gaining strength. As resistance training uses up a lot of glycogen, you should add 30 minutes of cardio training after it, as this would result in fatty acids being burned instead of glycogen. This is simply because there is no more glycogen left in the body to burn.

Therefore, the **4th rule** is; for starters, 1 hour every week is sufficient.

Chapter # 3: The Individual Target Heart Rate

Whether you're an elite athlete or a beginner, you should always stay within 90 to 110 percent of the target heart rate or THR.

The following is a method to calculate your target heart rate:

1. For beginners:

Target heart rate = ((220 – age) – RP) x 0.6 + RP

For example a 35-year-old starter with RP of 80 beats/minute would have a target heart rate of 143.

((220 – 35) – 80) x 0.6 + 80 = 143

Thus, for beginners it means that they should always be exercising at pulse rates in between 129 and 157 beats/minute.

2. For Intermediate:

A person is considered intermediate when he/she has completed a training of 6 months and is performing at least 2 cardio workouts every week.

The formula for them is:

Target heart rate = ((220 – age) – RP) x 0.75 + RP

For example a 46-year-old individual who has an RP of 60 would have a target heart rate of 146; his limit thus, lies in between 131 and 161.

((220 – 46) – 60) x 0.75 + 60 = 146

Both the formulas for starters, as well intermediate individuals, take the resting pulse into consideration, which makes it much easier to calculate the exact target heart rate. Slowly but surely, the body adapts to the changes and the RP decreases which indicates improved level of cardio fitness.

Chapter # 4: The Program

If you have no experience in engaging in any kind of cardio, then this is a good program to make up for it!

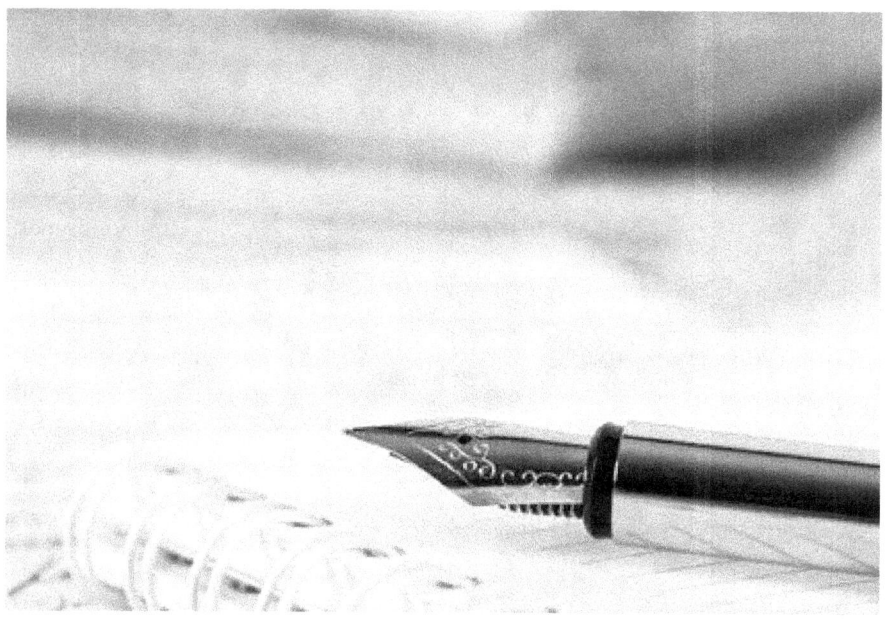

For the 1st Week:

Start off by walking 10 to 15 minutes every day; this isn't really that much if you think about it. Start by stretching the muscles of the legs after performing a warm up. Slowly increase your walking length every day and by the end of the seven days, you should have increased the walking duration to 30 minutes; remember to stretch after walking as well.

For the 2nd Week:

At the beginning of each of the walking sessions, walk for almost 15 minutes before starting to run at a slow speed. As soon as the pulse exceeds the prescribed target heart rate by more than 10 beats/minute, reduce your speed and begin walking again. Either walk or run for almost 30 minutes during this week, but never exceed the length of 45 minutes. Also remember to rest every other day if you feel too exhausted or sore from the previous day. If you feel energetic then keep on running every day.

For the 3rd Week:

Start by walking for at least 10 minutes followed by running. Keep watching your pulse and if it rises to a level greater than 10 beats/minute than the target heart rate, slow yourself down and start walking. Before giving up try to run at least 5 minutes.

For the 4th Week:

Start off the session by running at a slow pace; try your best to keep the heart rate below the target heart rate for at least 5 minutes. During the previous weeks, your body must have built up necessary stamina and you will most probably no longer need to walk.

For the 5th Week:

30 to 40 minutes of running would be required at least 3 times a week; the time given is for each session and not per week. Remember to stretch before, as well as after the run.

For the 6th Week:

This session is same as the fifth week, but during this week if you are able to reach the target heart rate for a time period of more than 45 minutes, then you would have to reduce the frequency to 3 days/week. If running for more than 30 minutes results in exhaustion then 3 training days a week are must.

During the whole program, the following rules must be kept in mind:

- Choose the time of the day to train according to your own personal needs; it may be night, it may be day.

- It is very vital that you stay within the 90 – 110 percent range defined for the target heart rate if you want to genuinely improve your cardiovascular fitness and cut fat instead of valuable carbohydrates. If you work out at too high a rate then you would only end up damaging yourself and develop a condition known as hypoglycemia, which is a condition that features extreme episodes of exhaustion due to very low levels of glycogen in the body. This condition can be easily avoided if the 110 percent limit is respected and followed.

- As soon as you wake up, it's best to measure your RP. A 15 second length of time to take the pulse reading is more than enough; all you have to do then is multiply the amount of heart beats by 4. During the first few days, the RP might even increase, but soon it must start to decline. If it keeps going higher, then add 1 – 2 days of rest in between the training regimen.

- Exercise will deplete the body of its liquid reserves, so it's best to keep yourself hydrated and drink after exercising.

Conclusion

The cardiovascular system is a complex combination of organs, veins, and other entities that make sure that the body gets proper nutrition. The epicenter of this system is the heart, which must always remain on if the body is to function. Therefore it is subjected to various hardships which must all be tackled systematically. One way to do so is through surgery or drugs, while the other one is through exercise. The later seems more promising, as it is a natural method with proven benefits. The material is pretty much self-explanatory and written in a transparent manner. If a healthy heart is what you want then you ought to follow it. With that said we wish you good luck in the training program and wish you good health. Remember to follow the instructions and not get into any take-the-pill solution or artificial diet that promises a million things upfront, but fails to deliver even one. That's all, Take Care!

References

https://www.fotolia.com/id/39676947

https://www.fotolia.com/id/41000500

https://www.fotolia.com/id/45319152

https://www.fotolia.com/id/41260110

https://www.fotolia.com/id/51802921

https://www.fotolia.com/id/52662791

Author Bio

Muhammad Usman is a distinguished medical graduate of Allama Iqbal medical college (AIMC). He is a professional writer who has been in the field for more than 4 years. During this time he has produced 10,000+ articles, blogs and eBooks on various niches related to diseases, health, fitness, nutrition and well-being. He is a regular contributor to several journals related to medicine and surgery. He is the editor of several journals and newspapers.

Check out some of the other JD-Biz Publishing books

Gardening Series on Amazon

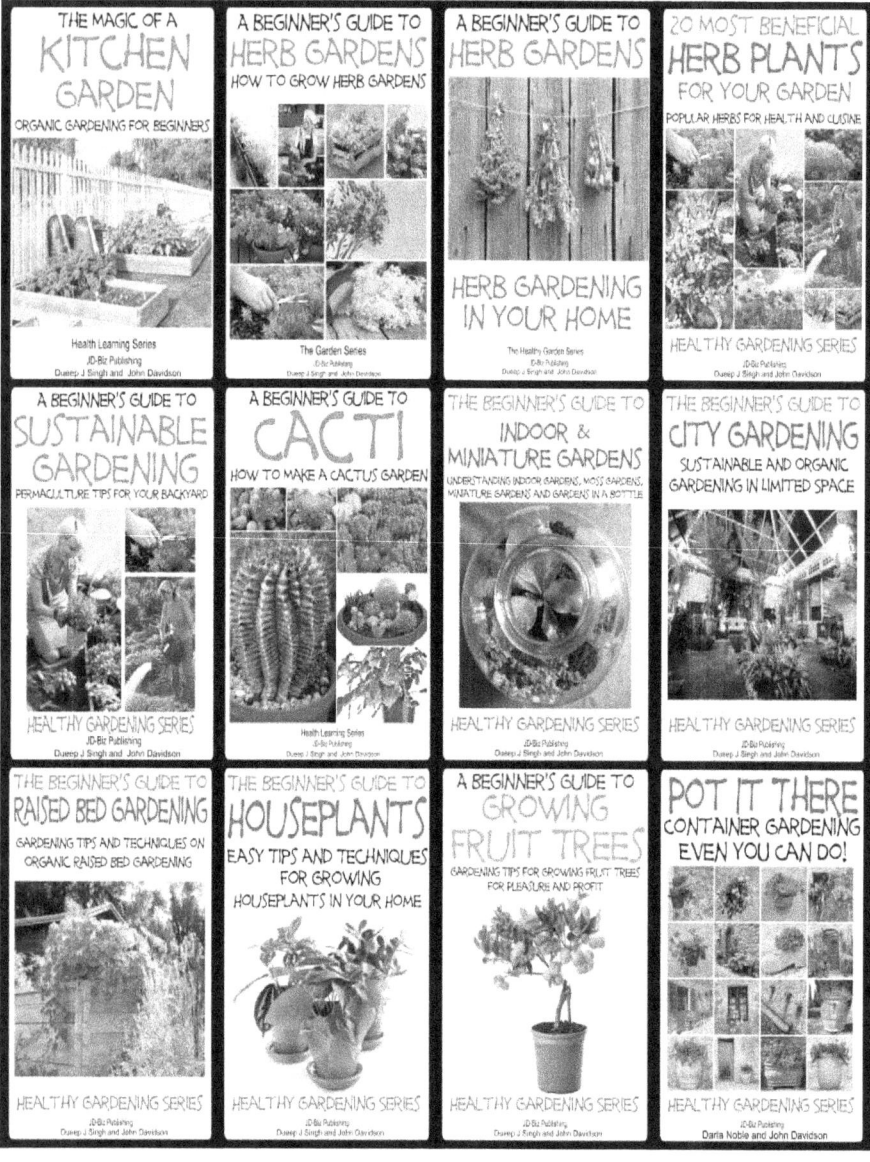

Health Learning Series

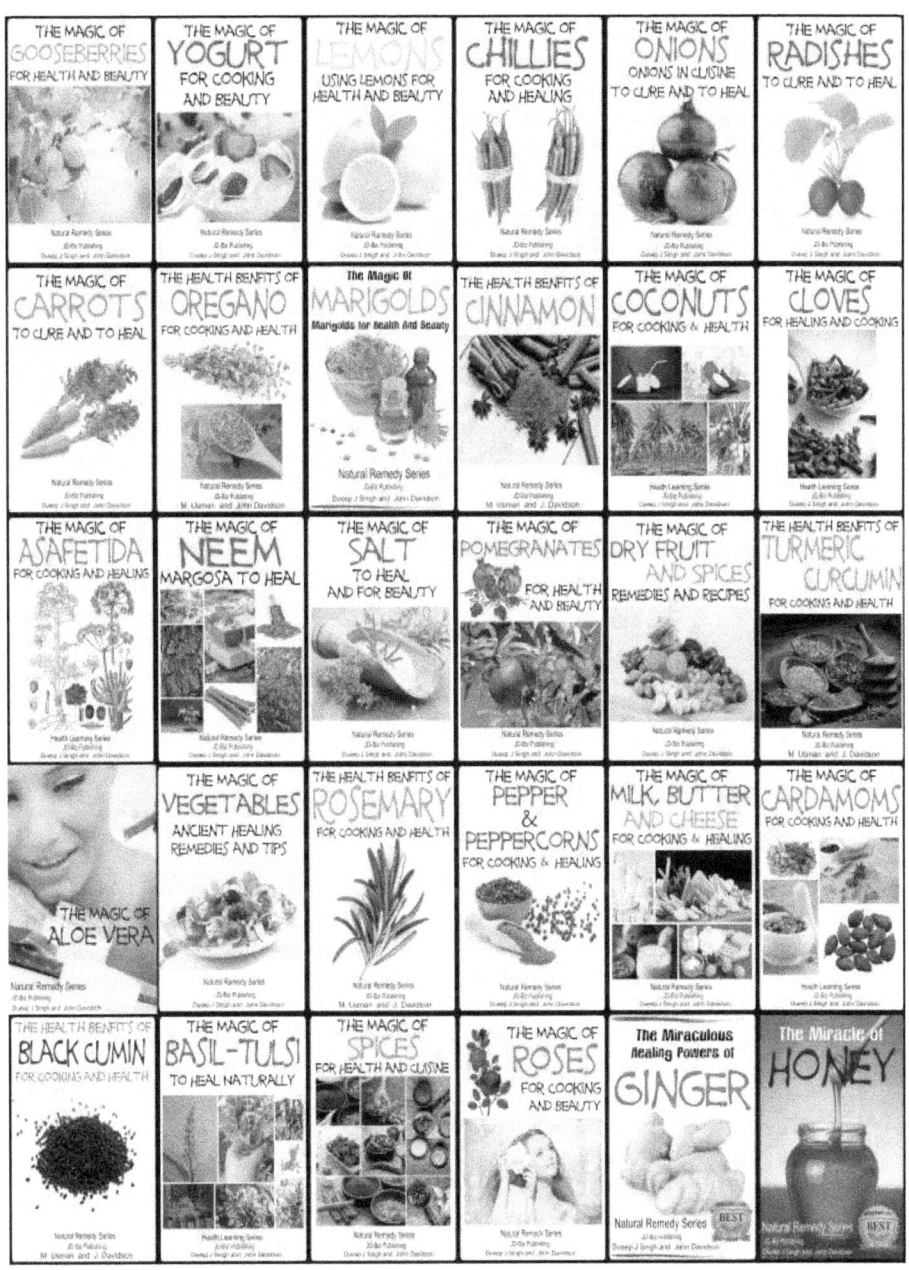

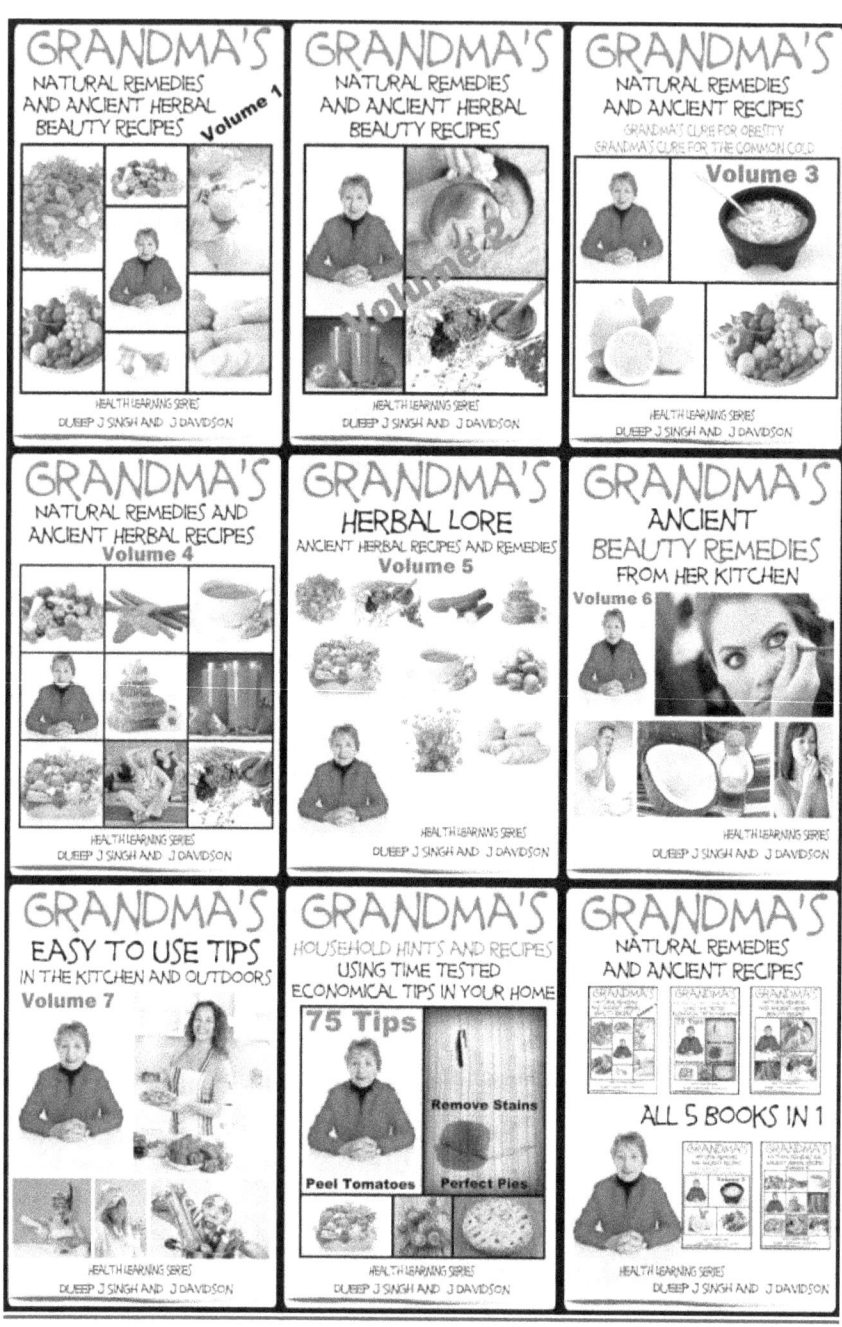

Country Life Books

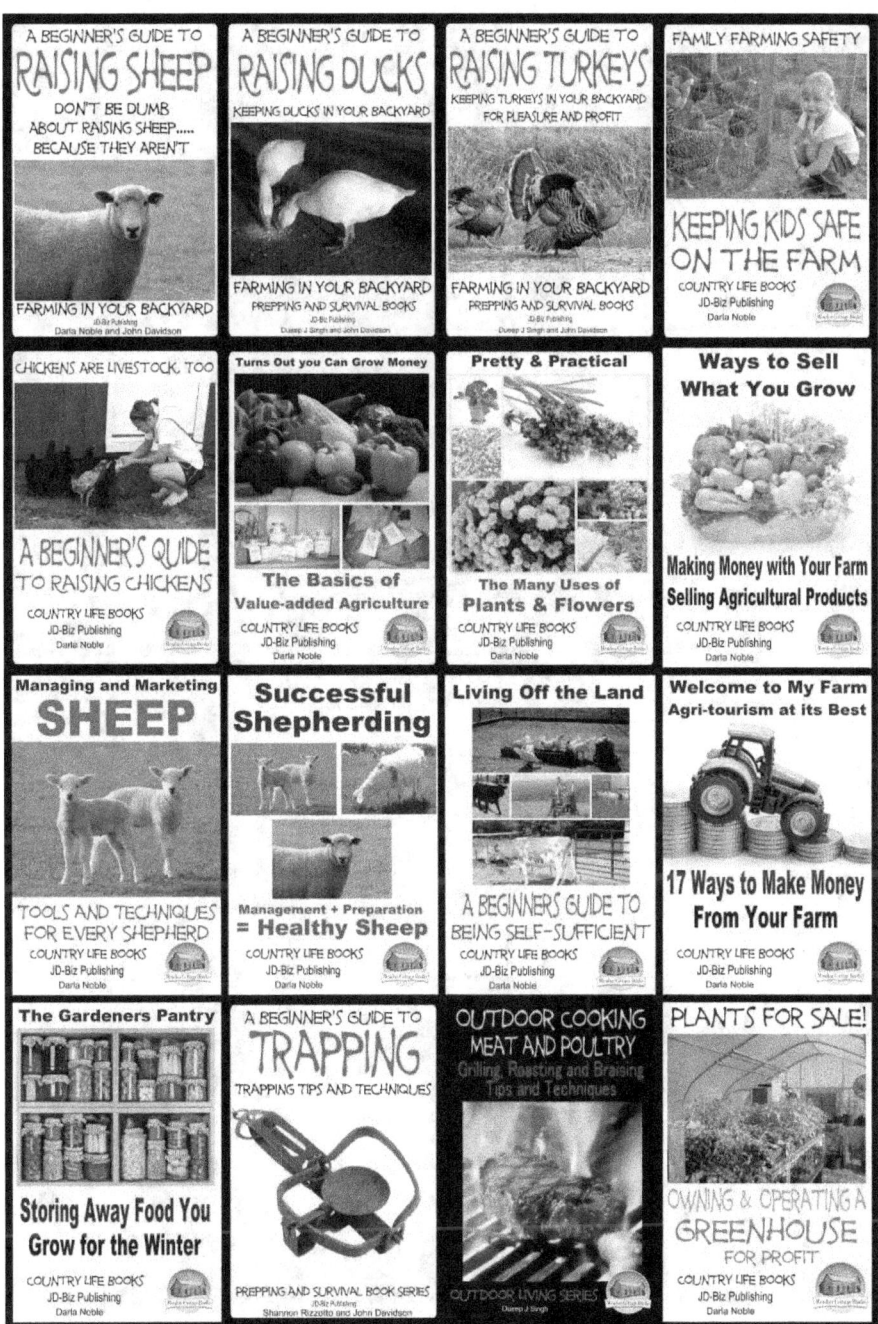

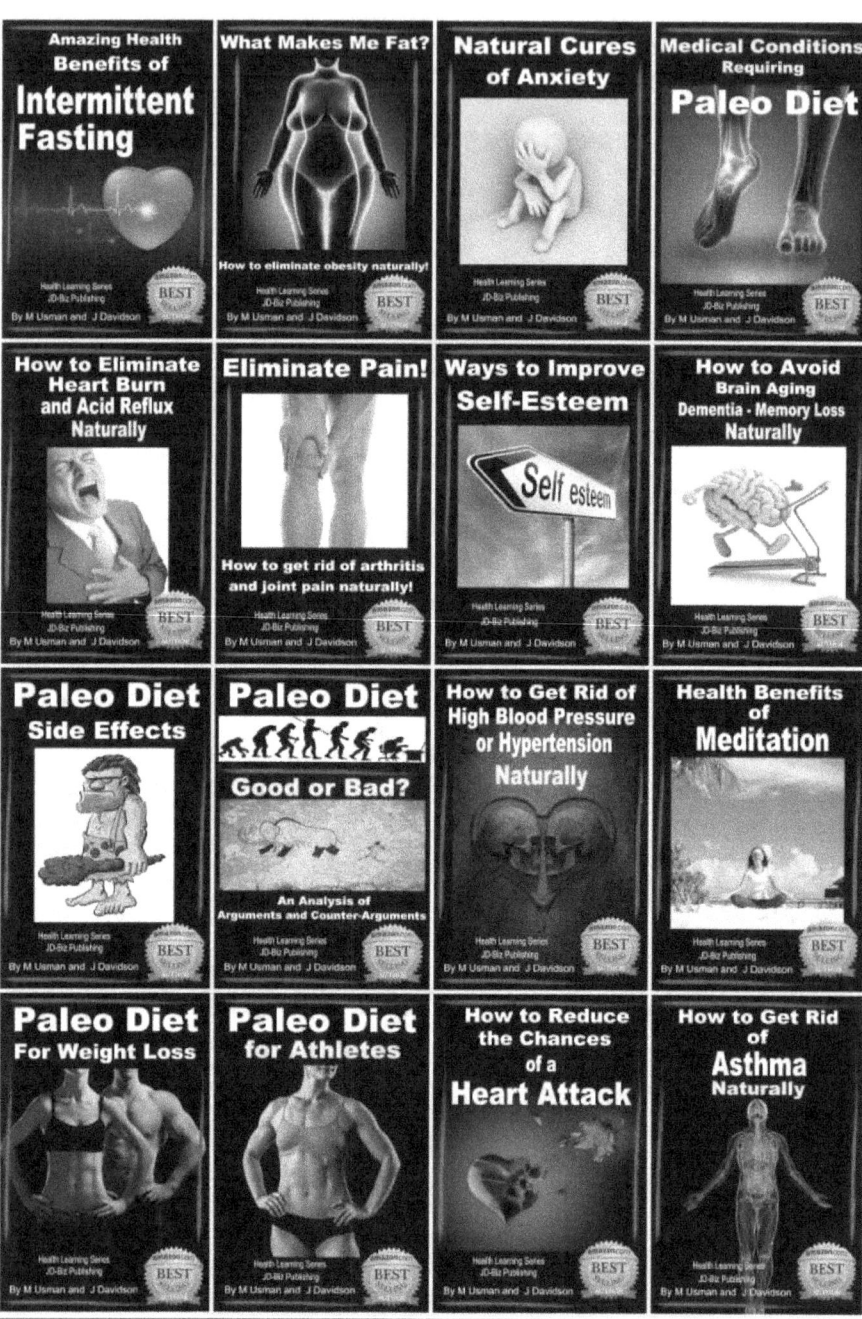

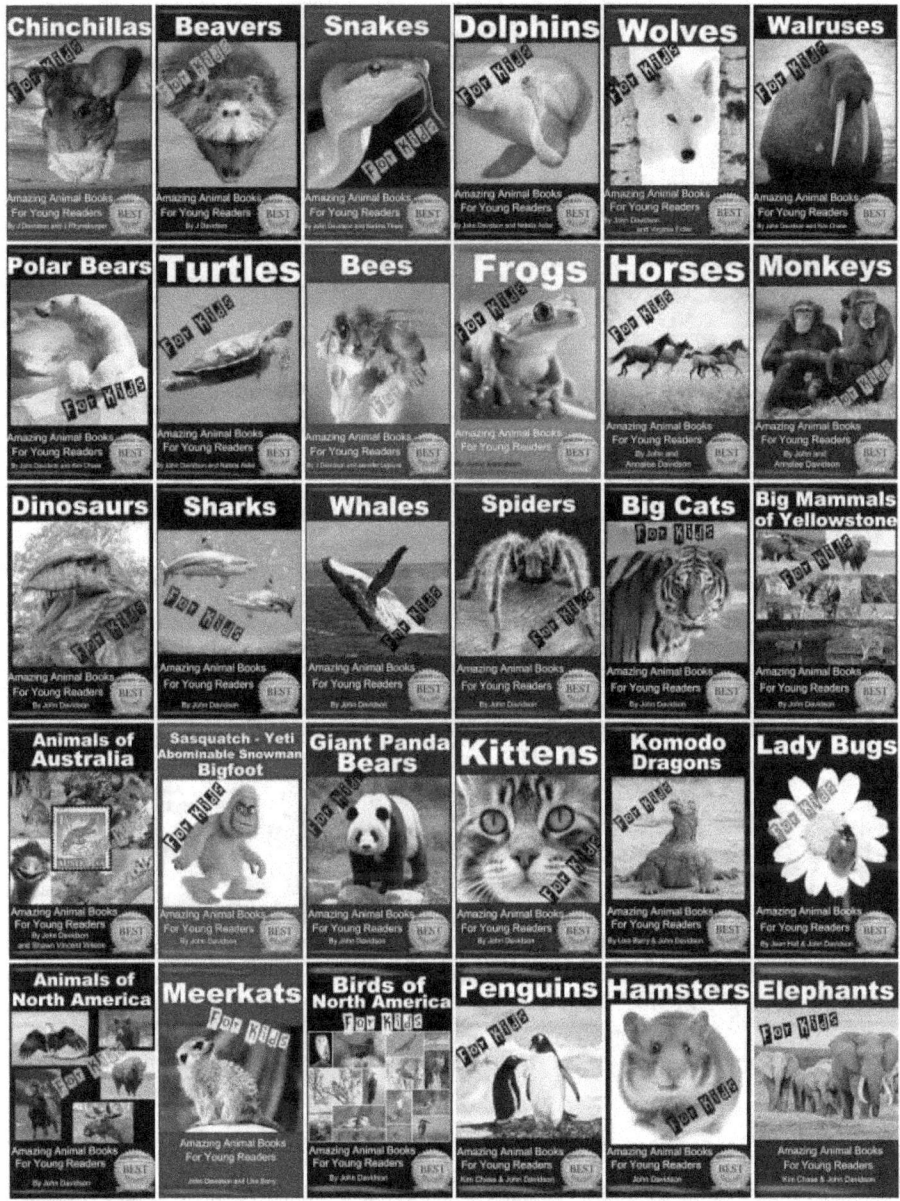

Learn To Draw Series

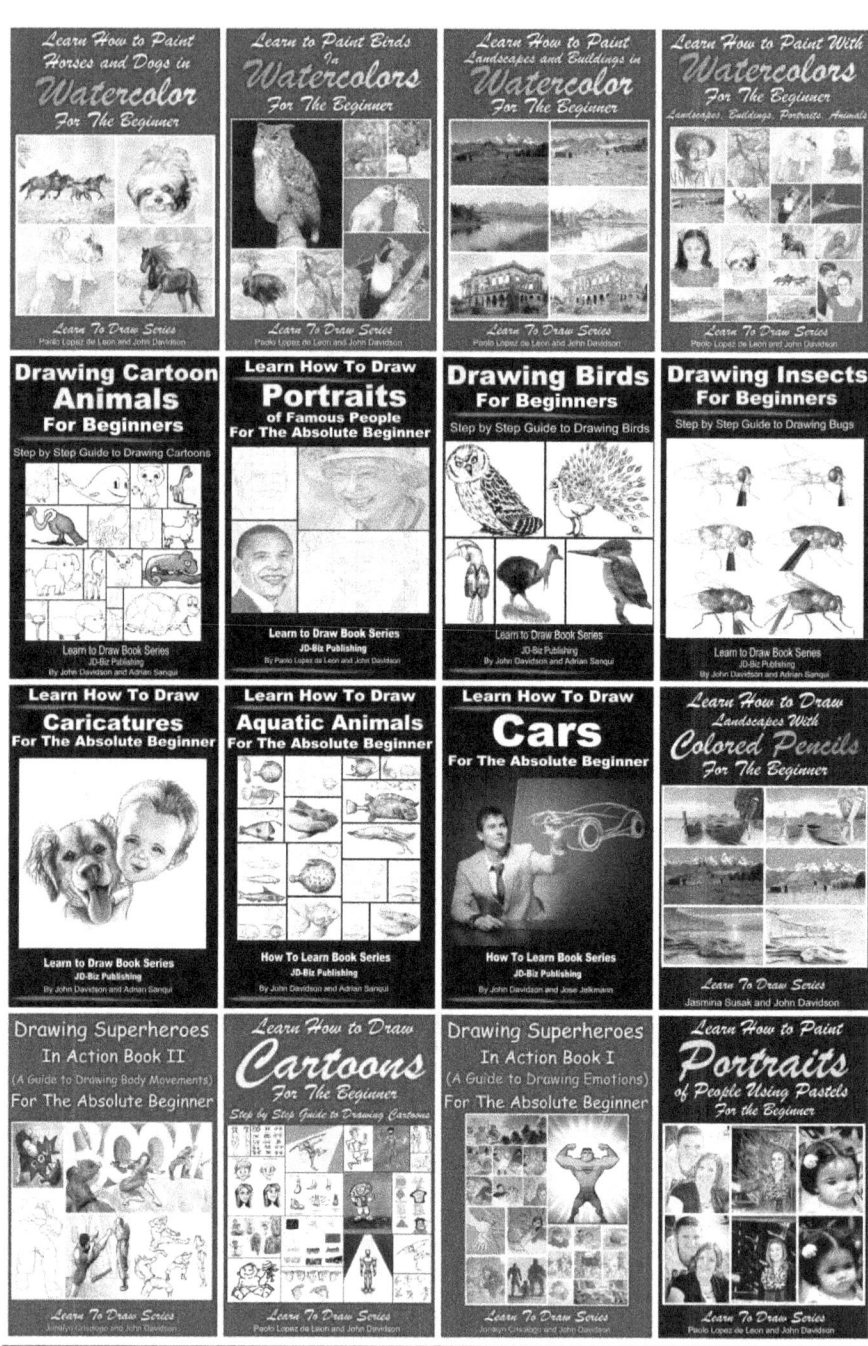

How to Build and Plan Books

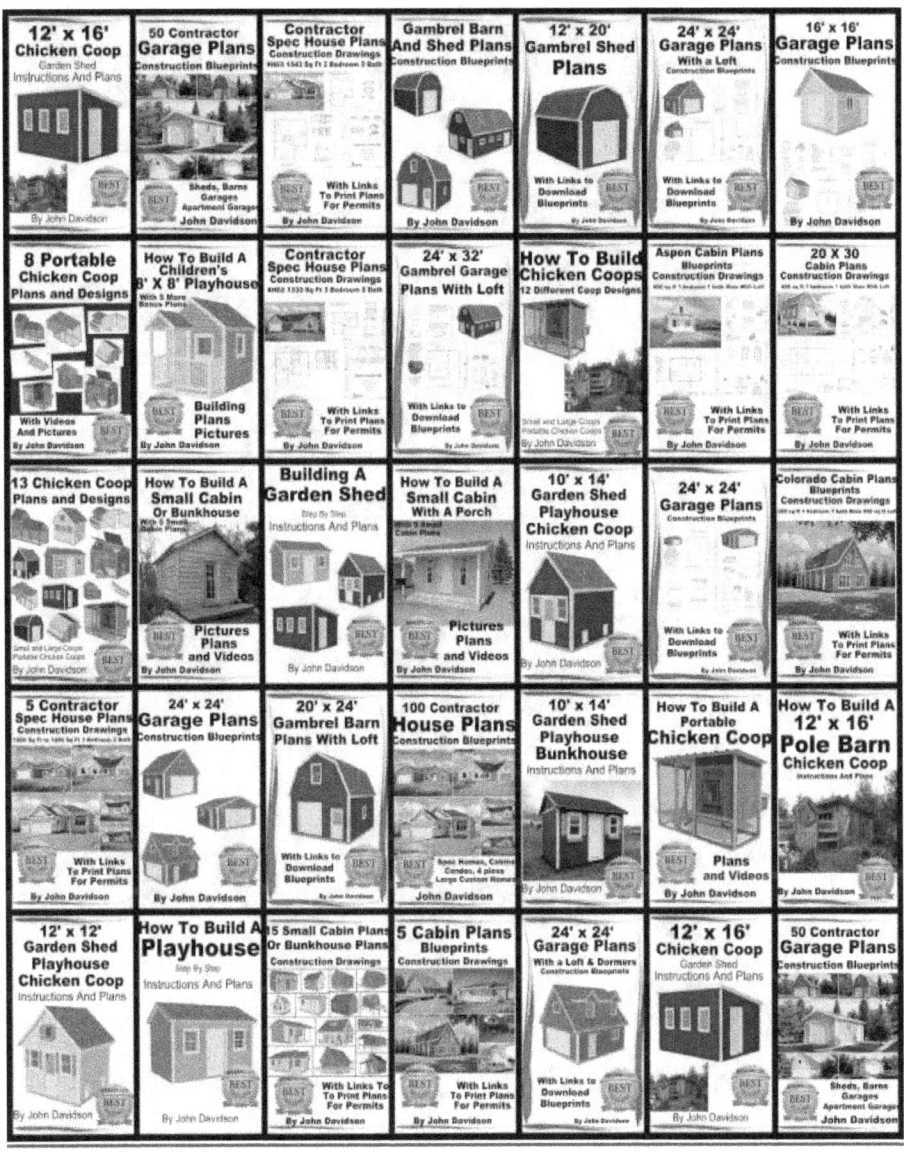

Entrepreneur Book Series

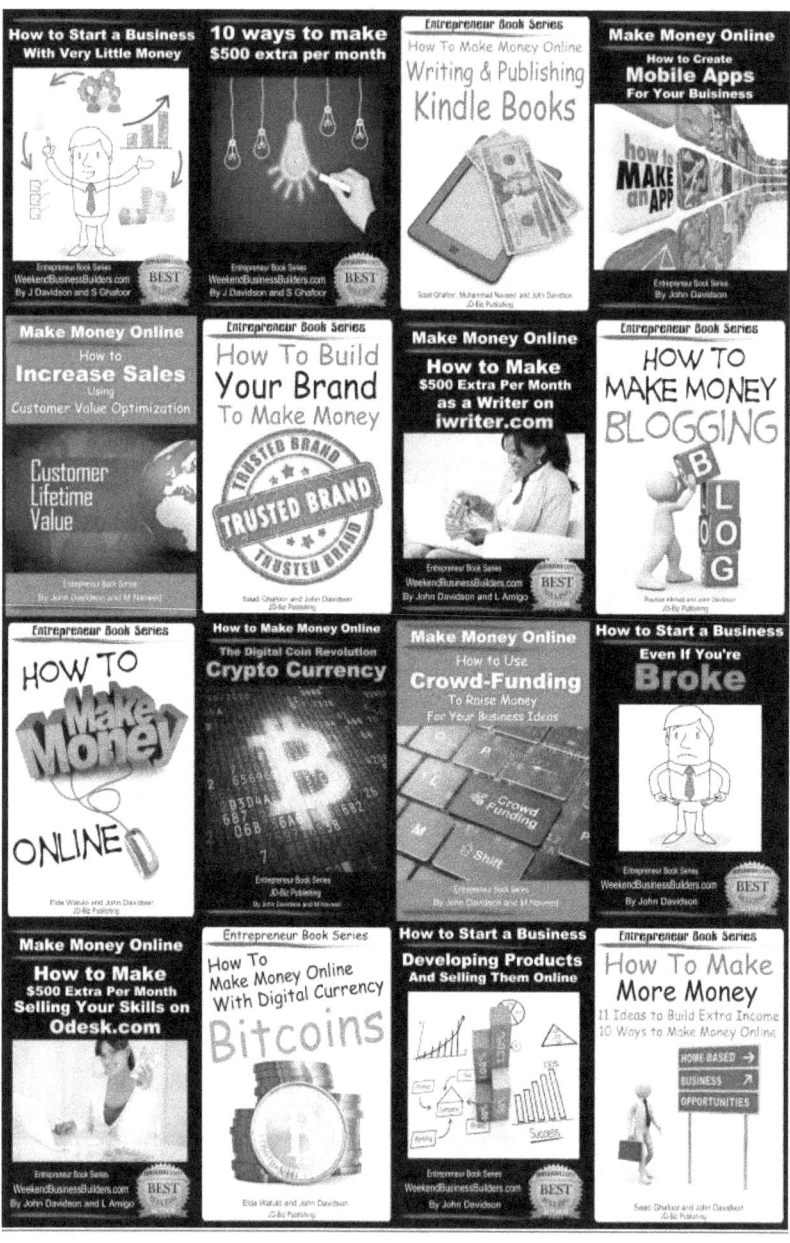

Our books are available at

1. Amazon.com

2. Barnes and Noble

3. Itunes

4. Kobo

5. Smashwords

6. Google Play Books

Publisher

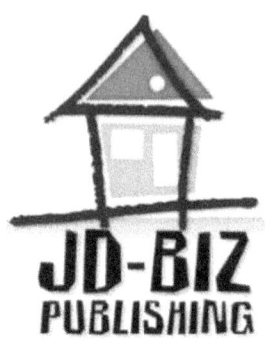

JD-Biz Corp

P O Box 374

Mendon, Utah 84325

http://www.jd-biz.com/

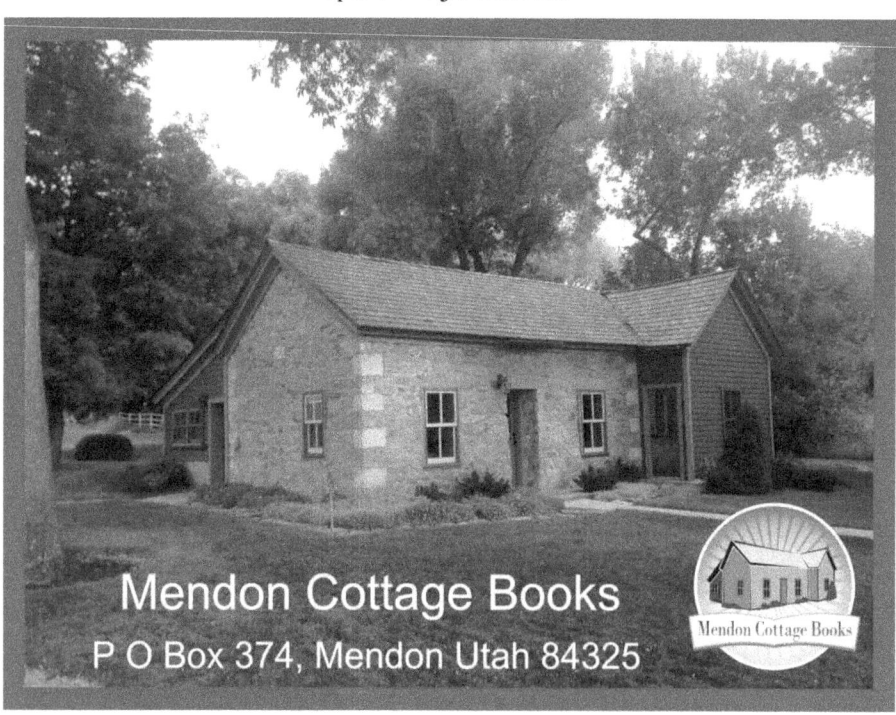

Mendon Cottage Books

P O Box 374, Mendon Utah 84325